The Ultimate Door Mounted Pull-Up Guide

The Last Piece of Home Exercise Equipment You'll Ever Need to Buy

John Carpinito

The Ultimate Guide to Door Mounted Pull-up Bars
The Last Piece of Exercise Equipment You Ever Need To
Purchase

Table of Contents

Introduction

You may have just purchased the last piece of home exercise equipment you will ever need. Home doorway pull-up bars are not only extremely effective for working your biceps and back muscles, but they can strengthen every muscle in your body. Just by changing your grips or the position of your legs, you can affect which muscles are engaged more and which engage less. It also affects which part of your body the workout is focusing is on. In this pamphlet I will break down everything from how to do your first pull-up, to how to work your whole body without needing to go to the gym. I hope you enjoy and get the most out of your new home fitness unit.

As a licensed physical therapist, I have always been a strong proponent of strengthening exercises as a way of preventing injury, and pull-ups are one of the best strengthening exercises you can do. Unfortunately, they are also one of the most difficult, so it is recommended that before you start you should consult with a physician to make sure that exercise and this specific type of exercise is right for you. Also, some of the exercises which will be listed below are extremely difficult to perform correctly and are meant for higher level athletes and need time to build up to. Always go slow and work your way up in a slow controlled time frame. You should also stop using this equipment if you start to experience any increased pain or feel any other symptoms such as very rapid heart rate, dizziness or nausea. Make sure to stretch and warm up appropriately before attempting to use this equipment because as we discussed it can be a very intense workout.

If you have never done a pull-up or chin up, I will walk you through how to get started. The first thing you should do is position yourself directly under the bar with your hands about shoulder width apart and facing away from you. This is a good starter position for a first pull-up. If you cannot reach the bar, stand on a step stool to get your hands up to the level of the bar. Once your hands are on the bar, grip it tightly, tighten your upper

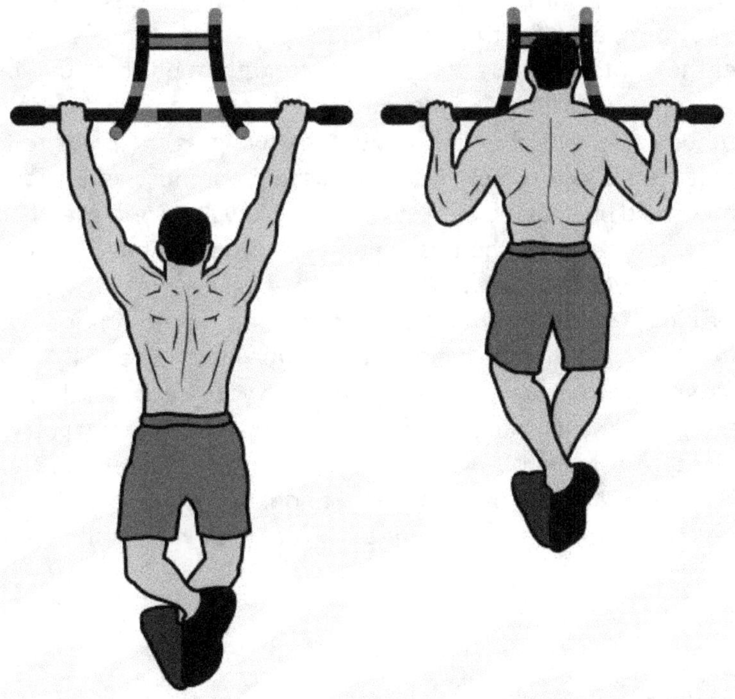

back muscles and lift your feet off the ground behind you. Now just hang there for a moment. When you are ready attempt to pull yourself up so that your chin clears the bar and your chest is touching or close to touching the bar.

You should be breathing in conjunction with the flow of the exercises. Exhaling on the way up and inhaling on the way back down. This will prevent injury due to holding your breath while exerting force into the pull-up. Once you have done this slowly lower yourself back down and repeat if possible. A good pace to perform the pull-ups at is a 2-3 second count on the way up and a 2-3 second count on the way down. This will prevent any jerky motions which will in turn prevent injury. Also, the slower and more controlled your pacing, the more muscle activity and muscle growth. Congratulations, you have just completed your first pull-up!

If you are not able to pull yourself up as described above, do not be discouraged. Pull-ups are one of the hardest exercises to perform, even for the most athletic of people. It takes time to get the right technique and enough strength to perform pull-ups properly. Two of the biggest mistakes people make when doing pull-ups are using their momentum or swinging their legs to try to lift their body up. This is dangerous for your muscles and joints and should be avoided as best you can. Slow and controlled body movements will be the best thing you can do to build strength and keep yourself safe. The second thing people do wrong is reaching their necks up over the bar when they are not strong enough to pull themselves all the way up with their arms. This is a great way to injure your neck and strain your back muscles. So, take your time learning and doing a pull-up correctly and you will get the most out of your workouts. In the next section I will describe which exercises you need to do, and which muscles you need to strengthen to get your body ready for your first pull-up.

Performing Your First Pull-up

When attempting to do your first pull-up you have to realize that even though the pull-up can work most of the muscles in your body, the most important ones that we need to focus on at the start are the biceps and the latissimus dorsi muscles and to a lesser extent your core muscles. Another thing to understand is that even though you have the strength in those muscles, you might need to re-educate them to fire appropriately. A pull-up is a closed-chain exercise and in order to do one, your muscles need to be trained to fire in a closed-chain manner. So, if you want to do some exercises on your own to prepare for this, but make sure to stick with closed-chain exercises.

For our purposes we will discuss 2 different methods to train your body to do a pull-up. These are by doing a modified pull-up or a negative pull-up. I have found that these are the fastest way to accomplish a first pull-up. I am going to show you how to do these in a simple easy manner so you can get those muscles strengthened appropriately.

First start with a modified pull-up. This can be done a few different ways but for now we are going to discuss a leg assisted modified pull-up. Just as the name says, you are going to use your leg muscles to help lift our body weight until your biceps and lats strong enough to do so on their own. Start by first putting a short chair or a stool under the pull-up bar. Stand on the stool so that your body is directly below the bar with your arms are straight up and holding onto the bar with a shoulder width grip. Now attempt to pull yourself up by using your arms to pull on the bar. As you are pulling use your leg muscles to push on the stool. The key is to use your legs as little as needed to get your body weight up to the bar. Then lower yourself back down. Each time you do a modified pull-up you should attempt to use your legs less and less until you no longer need them to assist you. If you do this over and over, you will notice it getting easier to get yourself up with your arms and back alone.

Another great way to train yourself to do a pull-up is to start with negative or eccentric pull-ups. In my opinion this is an even better way to train your body for its first pull-up. There is no better type exercise for strengthening and re-educating muscles than eccentric exercises. Research shows that eccentric exercises build muscles faster, more efficiently and reeducate muscles more efficiently than isometric or concentric exercises. To start, you stand on a stool and grab the bar with both arms about shoulder width apart. Then lift yourself up with your leg muscles until your chin clears the bar. Then take your legs off the stool and hold yourself up for as long as you can before slowly lowering yourself down in a slow controlled manner. The slower you can go, the quicker you will build and reeducate the muscles. We will discuss these in more detail further down in this pamphlet but that is the basics.

These two methods may appear similar, but they work your muscles in two completely different methods. One is a concentric exercise and the other is an eccentric exercise where the emphasis is on lowering yourself in a controlled manner. Both methods will help you strengthen the appropriate muscles and educate the muscle fibers to fire appropriately. Using a combination of both combined with some core strengthening exercises for added stability and leg control will give you the best results. It might not happen overnight, but you will be surprised at how well this method works. Once you have the first one under your belt, it is time to move on to some more difficult exercises.

Beginner Exercises

As I said above there are a lot of different exercises that can be performed just by changing your hand and leg positions. There are over 25 exercise variations that I have listed below to help you get the body you have always wanted, all while in the comfort of your own home. Each exercise will either focus on a new muscle group or will change the engagement ratio of the muscles which are activated, so you get a full body workout. I have broken up the exercises you can do while the bar is mounted on the door into 2 groupings by difficulty. A lot of them can also be combined to give you even more options for your workouts, such as close grip pull-ups combined with knees up pull-ups, etc. Also, some of these exercises are very advanced, so please go slow and work your way up accordingly. Let's get started!

Wide Grip: These are your basic beginner pull-ups, and the best exercises for getting that "V-shape" that most body builders and athletes want. To begin, stand directly under the bar and place your hands on the bar, with palms facing out and hands about 6-8 inches wider than shoulder width apart. Tighten your grip on the bar and tighten your upper back and trunk muscles and lift your feet off the floor so you are hanging there. Then slowly attempt to lift yourself by pulling yourself up until your chin clears the bar. Do not stretch your neck or raise your head to reach the bar. This will cause injury or discomfort to your neck area.   These are a great beginner pull-up and are great at focusing on the latissimus dorsi muscles in the back, the scapular rotators and to a lesser extent, the biceps muscles.

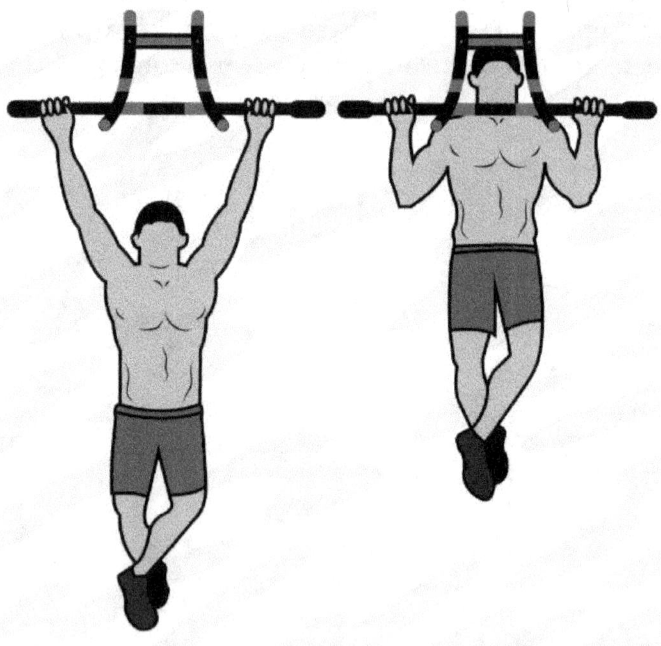

Close Grip: This variation is good for increasing range of motion (ROM) of the arms and shoulders which will in turn cause increased use of the muscles through that full ROM. They will therefore be more effective for increasing strength in those muscles. To start, stand directly under the bar and place your hands on the bar, with palms facing out and your hands about 4-6 inches apart. Tighten your grip on the bar and your upper back muscles. Then concentrate on your biceps muscles while you drive your elbows to the ground and attempt to pull yourself up until your chin clears the bar. These also focus on your inner lats, pectoralis muscles and lower traps.

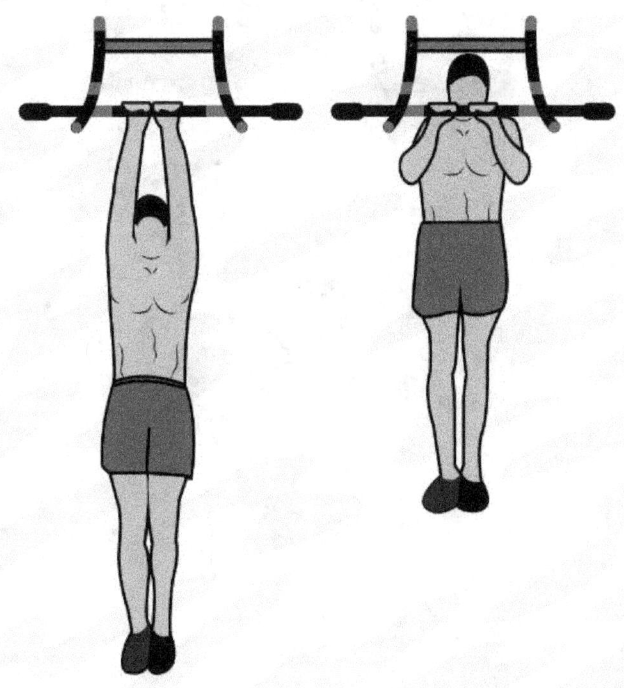

Neutral Grip: Utilizing the handles that come out from the bar, place your palms on the grips facing each other, and pull yourself up as previously. This style of grip will put the shoulders in a more neutral position and will therefore put less stress on the shoulder joint. It also allows the other elbow flexors other than the biceps to work in pulling you up. These include the brachialis and the brachioradialis muscles. Exercising these seldom used muscles will give your forearms extra pump and increased bulk.

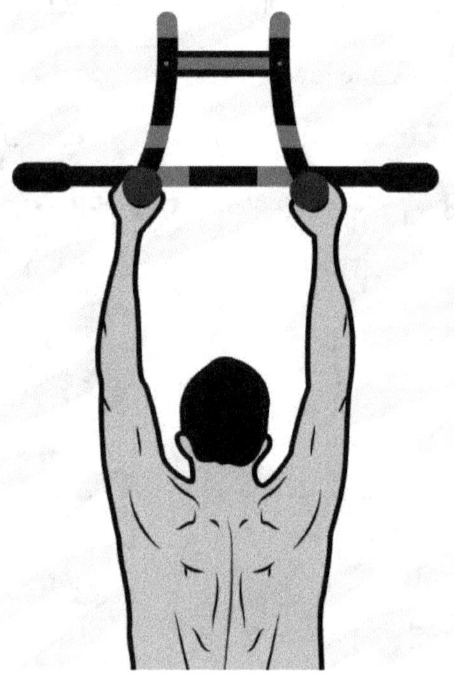

Chin Ups: Chin ups are slightly easier to do than pull-ups but allow for increased ROM of the shoulders, meaning that they will build strength faster and more thoroughly than pull-ups. Chin ups are performed with the palms facing in with your hands a little less than 8-12 inches apart depending on your body frame. Again, pulling yourself up until your chin clears the bar. These are amazing for the biceps, forearm flexors, and the mid and lower traps more than the lats. The pectoralis major and minor muscles are also activated more with chin ups as well as with narrow grip pull-ups.

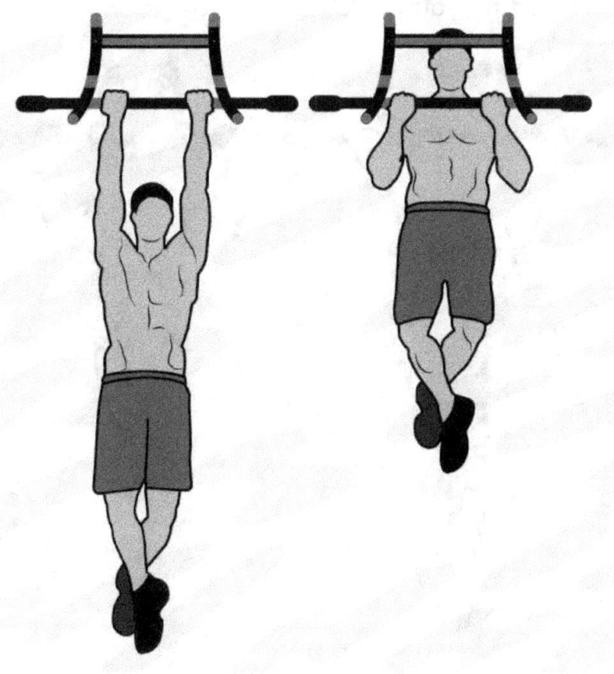

Mixed Grip Pull-ups: With mixed grip pull-ups you can vary your right-hand and left-hand placements on either side of the bar. This offers the same benefits as the grip being used, but the major benefit is that it helps to activate more trunk stabilizers and core muscles. This is because you need to keep yourself in a straight, neutral position while going up and down so your core muscles need to engage more to offset the different hand placement. Each different combination of grips can change which muscles and how much each of your core muscles are activated. Have fun trying different combinations and see which ones work best for you.

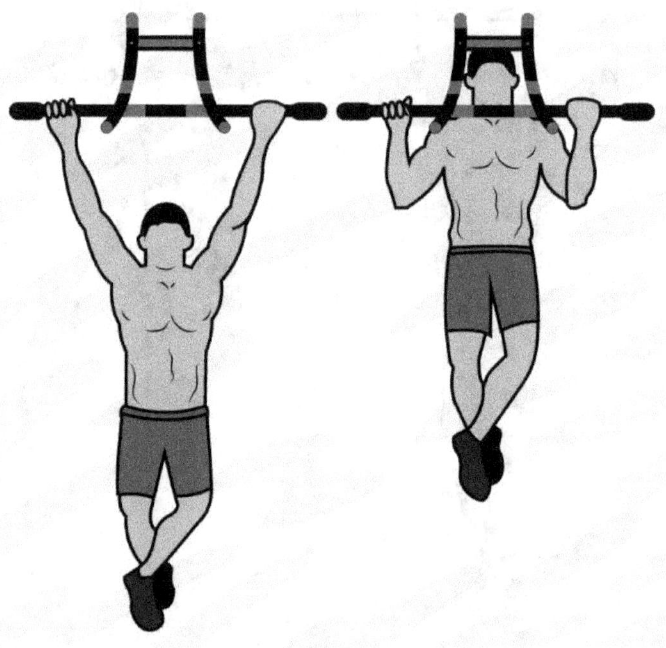

Negative/Eccentric Pull-ups: These are the ones we talked about in the section above for doing your first pull-up. They are also the most versatile of all the pull-up variations because eccentric muscle strengthening is not only effective for building strength, but it is also the best way to train your muscles for doing your first solo pull-up. As we discussed above if you are trying to perform your first pull-up this is the recommended method. To review, stand on a chair or stool so you can reach the bar, hold onto the bar with your hands shoulder width apart, and using your legs, push yourself up to a completed pull-up position. Then lower yourself down as slow as you can while maintaining control of your body and repeat. By doing this over and over it will build your arm and back muscles and it will re-educate them to fire in the manner most effective for performing a pull-up.   For those of you looking for increased strength, eccentric pull-ups can be done by doing a regular pull-up, then stop at the top and hold yourself isometrically. Then lower yourself as slowly as possible to build as much muscle as possible. The slower you lower yourself, the more muscle fibers which you will tear, and the more strength you will gain.

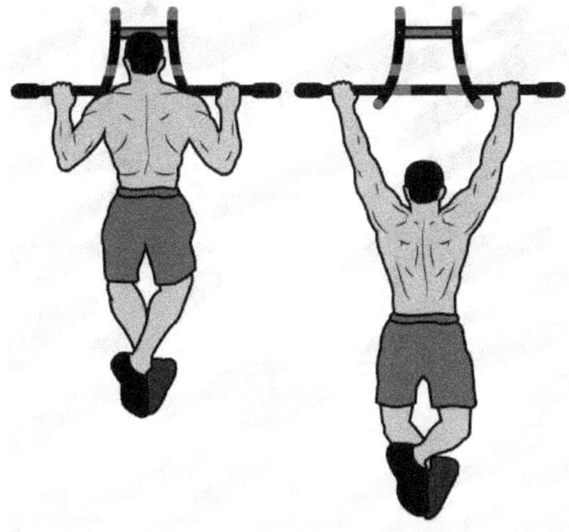

Hanging Shrugs: To perform these, grab the bar with a pull-up grip, shoulder width apart, and hang down with your arms extended. Then contract your posterior shoulder muscles so that your shoulder blades squeeze together and attempt to raise yourself upwards while keeping your elbows straight. This is a very slight motion which takes a little practice to get correct. Once perfected, you will notice a difference in your upper back and shoulder stabilizing muscles, mainly your rhomboids, serratus anterior and shoulder depressors.

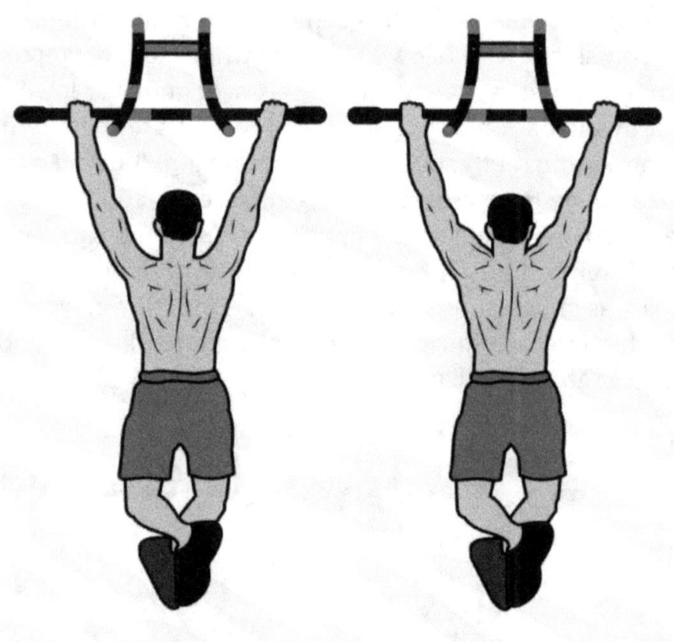

Dead Hangs: One of the most overlooked but effective exercises you can do with your pull-up bar are dead hangs. Just grab the bar with your favorite grip position and let your body just hang down. Not only does this increase your grip strength but it will increase the size of your forearms 10 times more than standard wrist curls. These are also great for strengthening your rotator cuff muscles which are one of the most important and most overlooked muscle groups in the upper body. Strong rotator cuff muscles help prevent injury and will keep the integrity of your shoulder joint intact when you are working larger muscle groups. A third advantage of dead hangs is spinal decompression. Hanging just 30 seconds to a minute at a time can help rehydrate your compressed intervertebral discs and decrease spinal nerve compressions. Pull-up straps can be used for this exercise if your goal is traction.

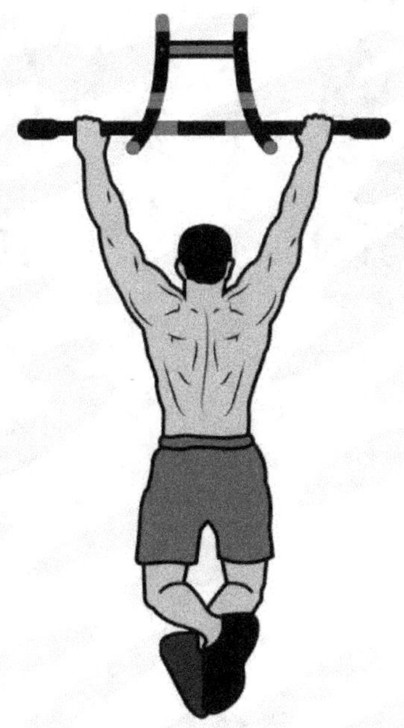

Hanging Forearm Curls: Speaking of increasing the size and strength of your forearms, these insanely effective exercises are amazing. They start out just like dead hangs, but with your hands facing away. Then attempt to curl your wrists forward while keeping your elbows straight. These are one of the best forearm strengthening exercises you can do. Every rep feels like your torturing yourself, and your forearms will never be the same.

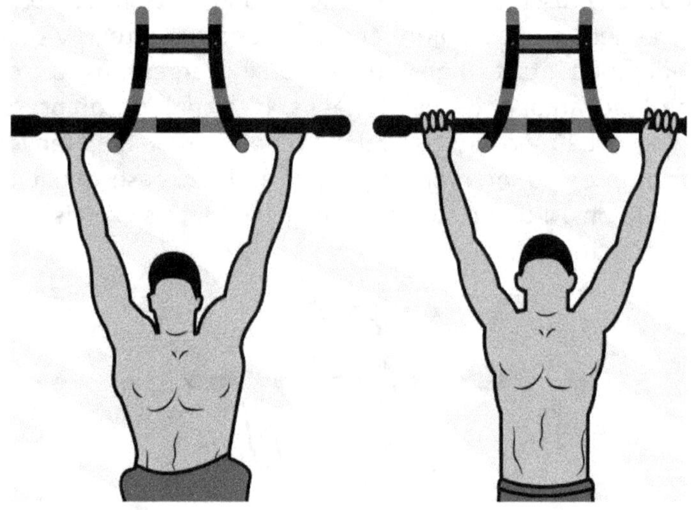

Pull-ups with Legs Behind: Leg position can be a big determining factor to which muscle groups get strengthen during a pull-up. When you move your legs behind you, your center of gravity changes and is pushed posteriorly. This means that you will be getting increased activation of your posterior spinal muscles when doing a pull-up. These include the erector spinae, intervertebral muscles and increased activation of your gluts and hamstrings. The further back you can get your legs, the more you will change the muscle activation.

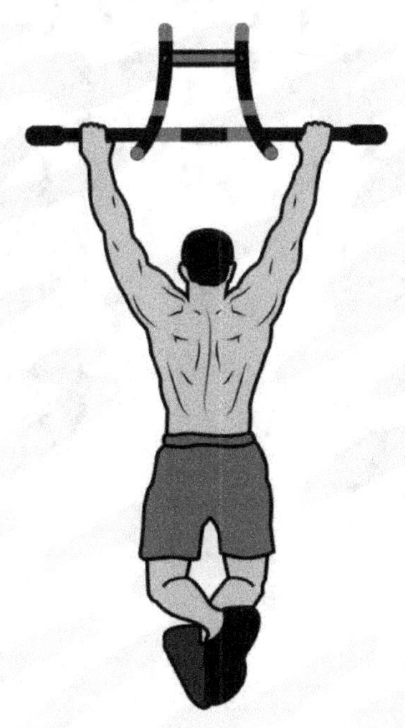

Pull-ups with Legs in Front: When your legs are positioned in front of your body, your center of gravity is moved anterior, meaning that you will be activating your abdominal and pelvic stabilizers more. There are many different variations of this that we will discuss in the advanced exercises section. Just putting your legs slightly forward will be a less difficult advanced variation of those exercises.

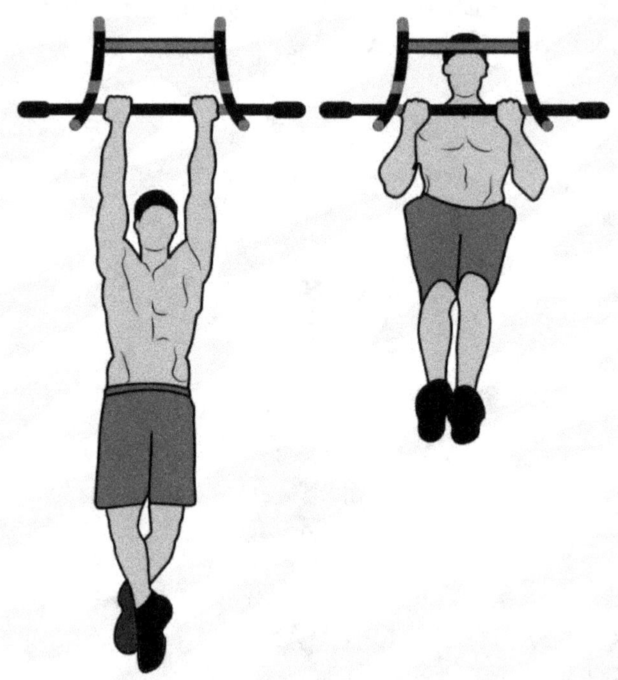

Advanced Exercises

The next set of exercises we will discuss are much more advanced and should be approached with caution. Most of them require a strong core and a high level of endurance in your upper body muscles. Building up to these is something you will need to work towards slowly and carefully. But if you are consistent with your workouts, you will be doing the hardest of them before you know it and you will be well on your way to the body of your dreams.

Pull-ups with Knees Up: These are a lot harder than they look and may take a little practice to perform properly. They are also the first in a long line of core strengthening exercises that you can perform with your pull-up bar. Just grab the bar in your favorite pull-up position and lift your knees up towards your chest. Hold them in that position by tightening your core muscles while you do a pull-up. These work just about every muscle in your body, with increased emphasis on your lower abdominals and pectorals.

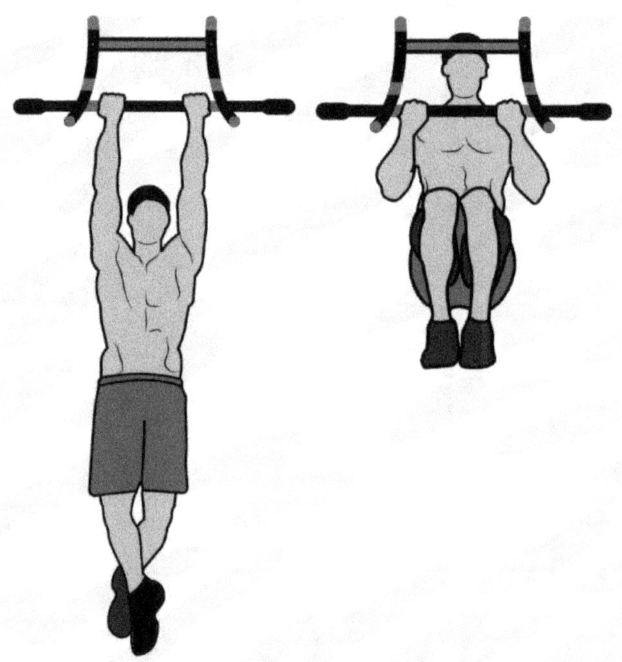

Single Arm Pull-ups: Start by grabbing the center of the bar with one hand, probably your most dominant arm, and then grab that wrist with your opposite hand and pull yourself up using both hands. These are a great variation to help increase grip strength mainly, but also shoulder stability, and core stability. The reason they work so well to increase shoulder and core stability is because by grabbing the bar with only one arm, your core muscles and shoulder muscles need to activate more to keep your body in alignment.

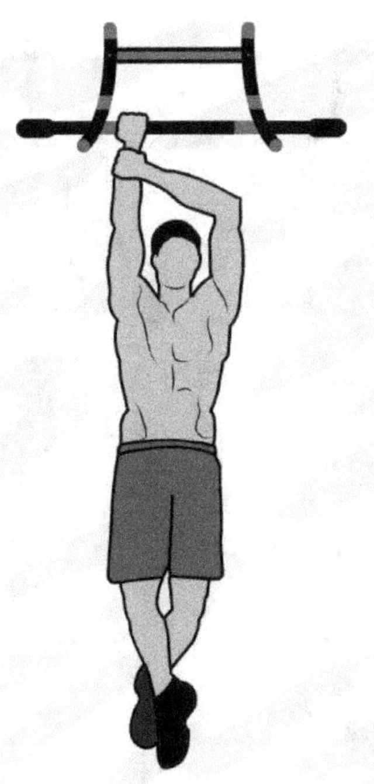

Towel Grip Pull-ups: Using two rolled up hand towels, one wrapped over each side of the bar, grip them with your hands and pull yourself up. This is another great exercise to increase grip strength and explode your forearm muscles. Shoulder stability muscle activation is also increased due to the lack of stability of the towels on the bar, forcing the shoulder stabilizers to do more of the work. If you thought your forearms were working hard with some of these other exercises, wait until you try a few of these.

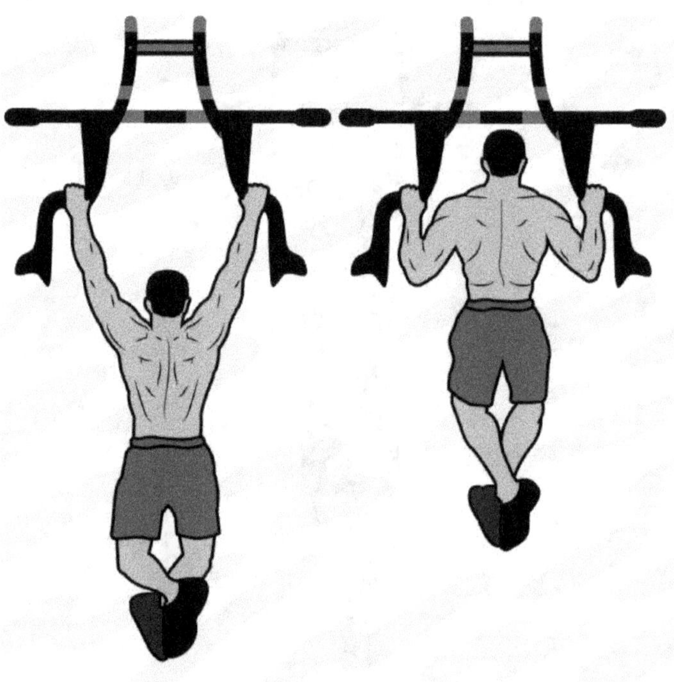

Weighted Pull-ups: These are self-explanatory, but extremely difficult to do. Just wrap a weight around your waist or legs and perform a pull-up. The main thing to keep in mind when doing a weighted pull-up is where you place the weight. If you place the weight in front of you, it will cause a greater activation of your anterior muscles such as your abdominals and if you put it behind you it will engage the erector spinae and posterior back muscles more. The type and size of the weight you use is up to you but be careful not to overdo it unless you have someone to spot you.

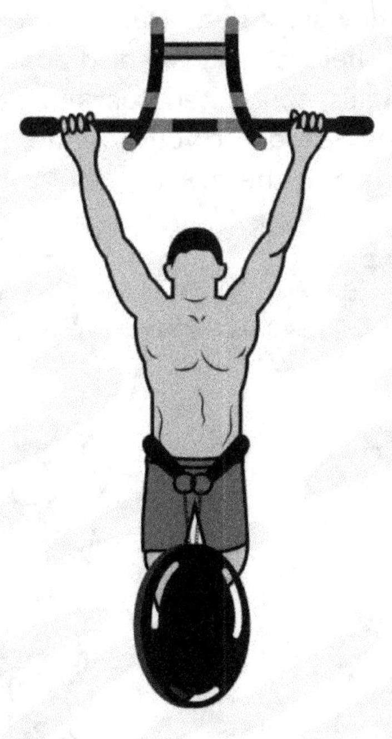

Hanging Knees Raises: Grab the bar in a close grip, chin up position or use arm straps to hold up your body weight. This exercise as well as most of the abdominal exercises below are best done with arm straps to hold your body weight, so your grip does not give out before your core muscles get fatigued. Then try to contract your abdominals and hip flexors and lift your knees so that the tops of your knees touch your chest if possible, then lower your knees back down slowly. These are a great exercise to increase engagement of the lower abdominals and hip flexors. Plus, they are a good training exercise for the next few exercises listed below. You can also do a bicycling motion with your abdominals contracted for another more difficult option, or to add some cardio to your routine. You will want the pull-up straps when doing these.

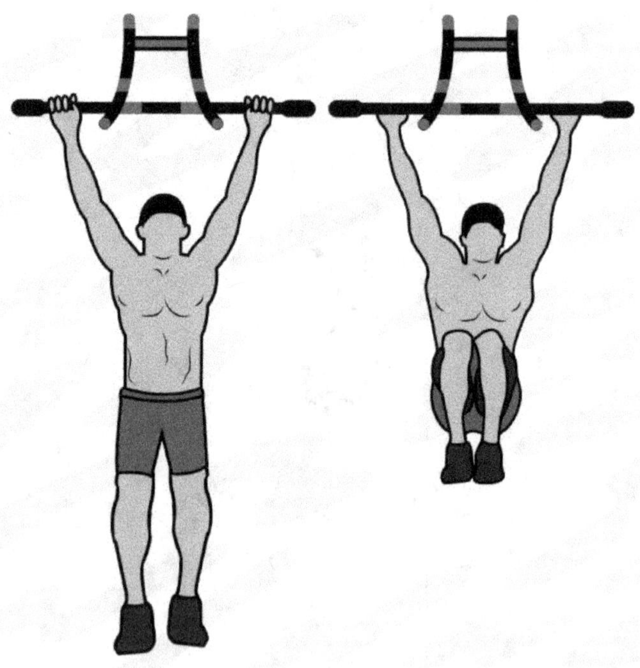

Hanging Leg Raises: Same as the hanging knee raises, but you are keeping your knees straight while you lift your legs together, bending at the hips. These are much harder to do than the knee raises because you are increasing the lever arm by keeping your legs straight, making the abdominals work extremely hard to lift your legs, and to eccentrically lower them back down in a controlled manner.

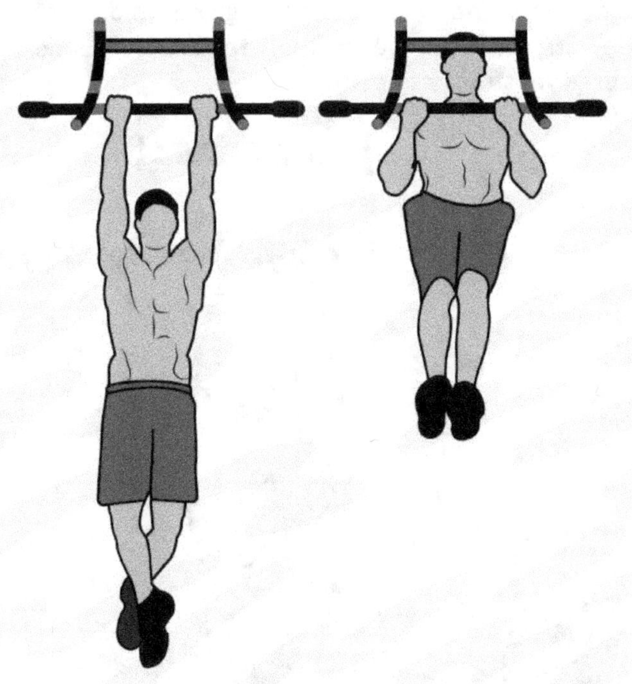

L Hangs: Now we are really getting into the difficult abdominal and core strengthening exercises. These are performed the same way as the leg raises, but instead of lowering and raising your legs, you hold them straight out so your body is in an L shaped position for as long as you can. The key with doing these properly is to make sure your back stays straight and does not arch forward while holding your legs up, and to make sure you continue to breathe while performing the hold portion of the exercise. Try to hold the position for 5-20 seconds to start. Again, use arm straps as needed.

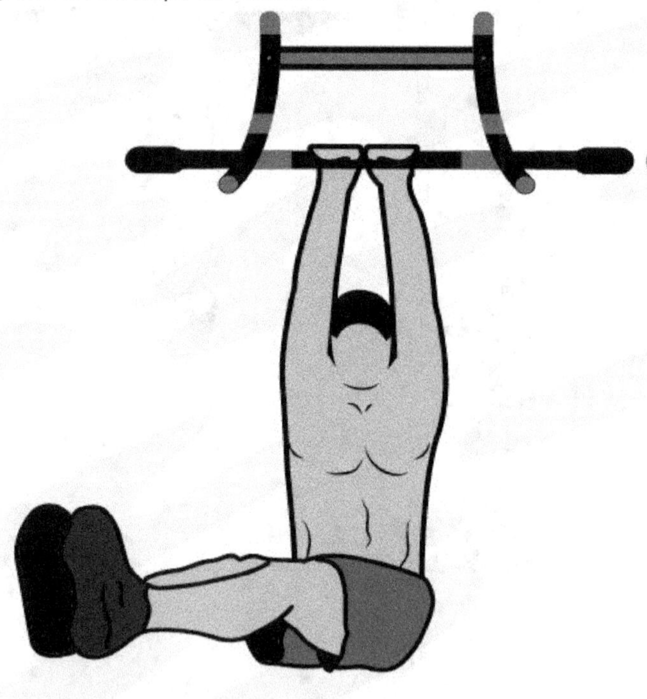

L Hangs with Rotations: These are the same as the L Hangs but when you get to the top of the hold position, you rotate at your pelvis so your legs turn from side to side while in the L hang position. This engages not only the abdominals but the internal and external oblique muscles, giving you a full core workout.

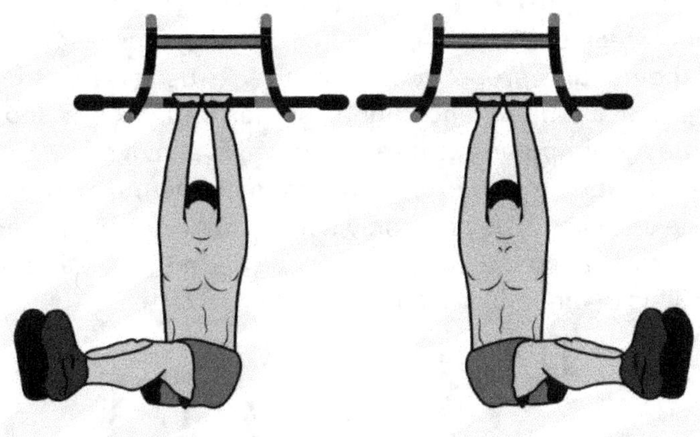

Toes to Bar: This exercise is just as the name implies. To perform it, you grab the bar tightly and pull your body towards it while you attempt to curl your abdominals and finally attempt to kick the bar. Once you get to the to the top and your toes touch the bar remember to not just let your legs fall back down quickly as it can cause a negative momentum and increased back pain. Another thing to watch for when performing these is to not let your momentum propel you and your legs up towards the bar. This is called kipping and cannot be performed on a doorway mounted pull-up bar because it can come unhinged and fall to the ground due to the quick changes in momentum. These are no joke and should be done only when you have built up enough muscle strength and endurance from perform them in a slow and controlled manner. Proceed at your own risk!

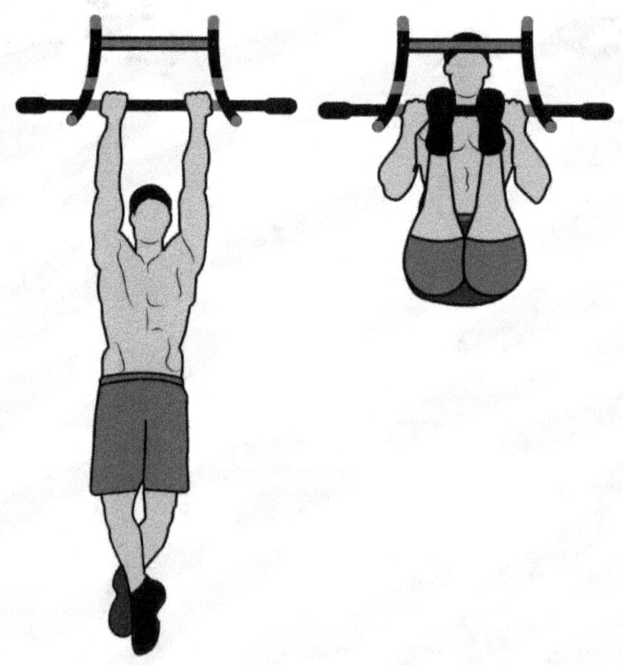

Side to sides: With hands facing out and slightly wider than shoulder width apart, do a pull-up until your chest is touching or close to touching the bar. Then hold that position and begin to move your body from side to side at a slow even pace. This is a challenging exercise to perfect but is very gratifying when you can do it correctly. It is an extremely effective exercise for strengthening the shoulder rotators and stabilizers as well as the pectoral muscles. It also is a great isometric strengthening exercise for your biceps and lats.

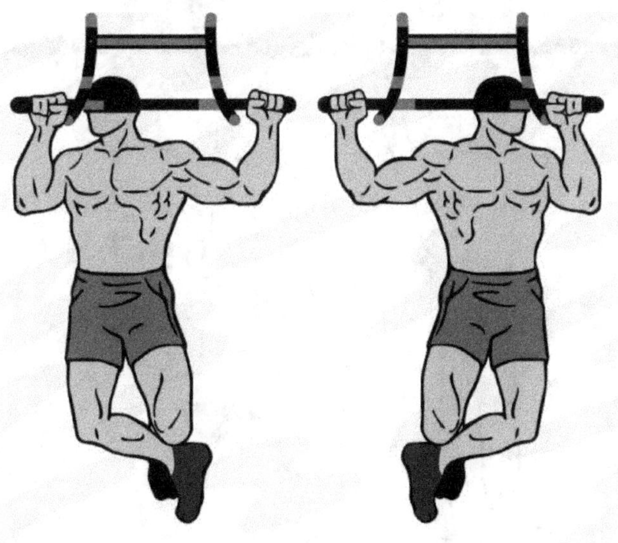

Knee side raises: These are another difficult exercise to perform but will give you a great abdominal and oblique workout. Hold the bar or place your arms into the arm straps then bend and lift your knees at an angle and rotate your trunk so that your knees are moving diagonally towards your opposite elbow. Then lower back down to the center with legs straight and lift and bend to the opposite side. Continue to repeat in a rhythmic motion from side to side.

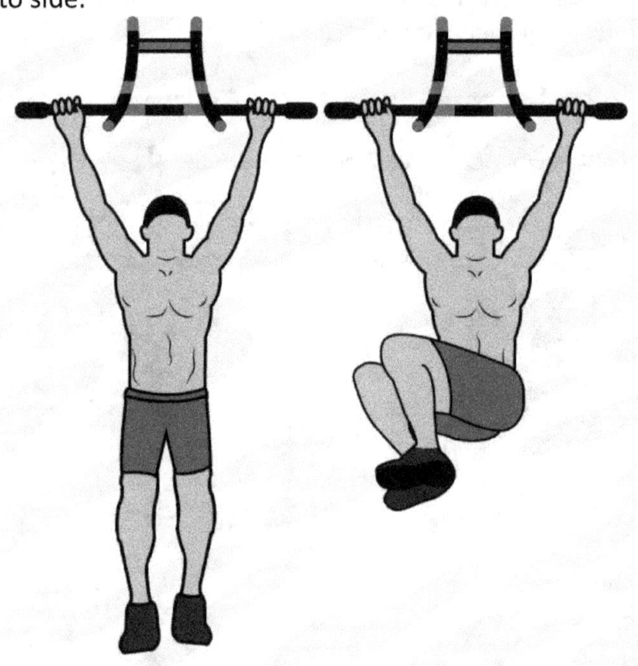

Exercises with Bar Not Mounted

Next, I will discuss a few bonus exercises that you can do with your doorway pull-up bar when it is on the floor. These exercises are a great way to work on muscles that you will need later when performing the pull-up exercises listed above. They are also good for adding a change of pace to your pull-up workout routine. One of the few muscle groups that does not get a great workout with pull-ups are the triceps. Some of these exercises are a great way to incorporate your triceps muscles into your home workout routine.

Also, with all the following exercises, as we already discussed with the pull-ups, breathing and pacing are extremely important for injury prevention and muscle growth. Exhaling while contracting your muscles and inhaling during the rest period of the exercises is the best practice. As with the pull-ups, pacing should also be 2-3 seconds in each direction, with no jerky or violent movements. For a negative or eccentric strengthening option, slowly count 5-10 seconds while coming back down, or during the elongating portion of the exercise. Lastly, remember not to lock out your elbows when you straighten out your arms. This is another easy way to injure yourself.

Sit ups: Doorway pull-up bars make the whole process of doing sit up much easier because they can provide the stability you need at your feet, so you can focus more strength into using your abdominals. First place the bar on the opposite side of an open doorway so the long part of the bar is blocking it from sliding forward. Then lie down on your back on the opposite side of the doorway with your hands behind your head or across your chest and slide your feet under the bar as in the picture so your feet cannot slide back. The key with sit ups is to not flex your neck or move your head at all. Once your head is stabilized, tighten up you core muscles while keeping your spine completely straight, and sit up so that your elbows move towards your knees, then lower yourself back down slowly. Sit ups are great for working your hip flexors and upper abdominal muscles. You can add rotations to incorporate your obliques as well.

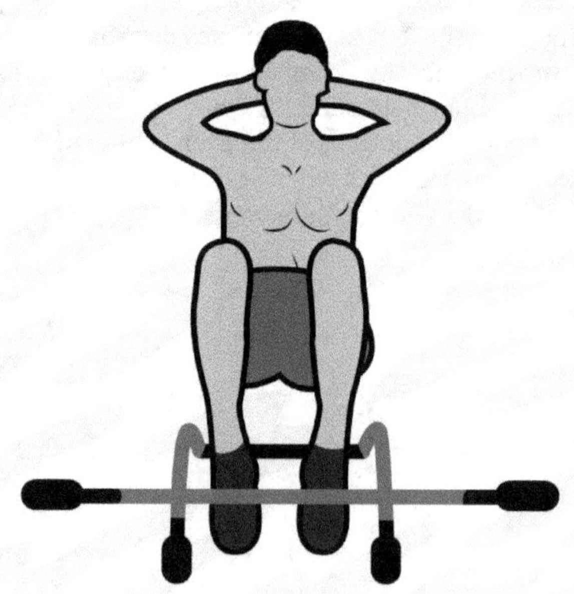

Crunches: The set up for crunches is similar to the set up for sit ups, but instead of sitting your whole upper body up and flexing at your hips, try to just raise your shoulders off of the floor without flexing your head forward. A great trick for doing this correctly is to imagine a string that is attached from your nose to you the ceiling directly above you. Then imagine that string pulling your nose straight up. That is the direction you want to move your head and shoulders but without pushing your head forward. Also, no holding your breath during this exercise or it can be dangerous to perform. These are great for working your lower abdominals to get you ready for some of the harder exercises we discussed above.

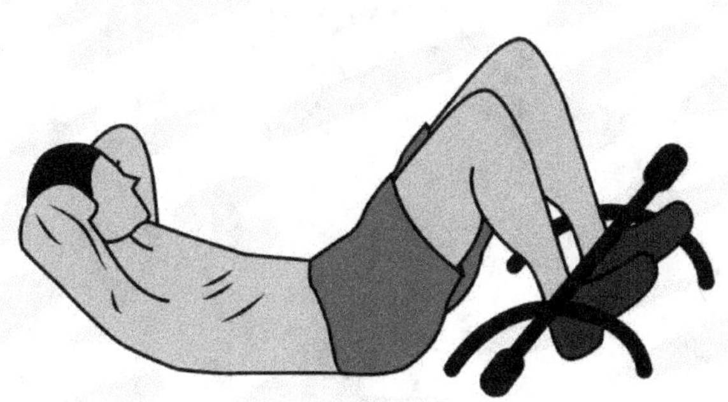

Dips: Place the bar on the floor so that the round part of the bar is facing up. Sit as close as you can to the bar so that your back is to the bar. Then reach back and grab the top of the rounded portion of the bar and push yourself up so your elbows are straight. Your legs can either be straight with your heels on the floor or have your knees bent with your feet on the floor. If you keep your legs straight, they will be more difficult than if your knees are bent. Start with your knees bent and progress to having your legs straight. These are both great for strengthening your triceps and pectorals mostly, but do not be surprised if you feel your abdominals and back muscles working as well.

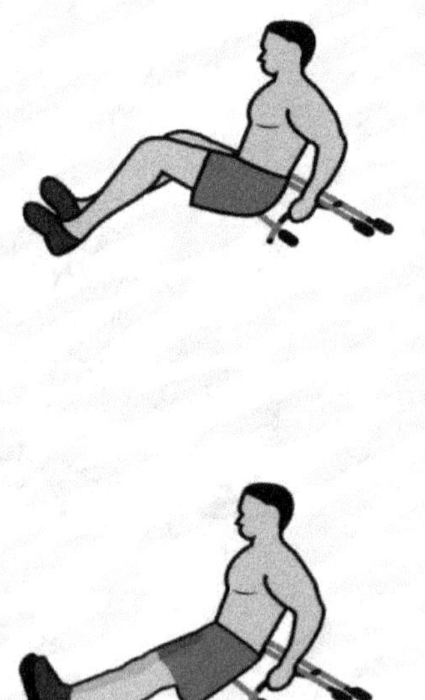

Wide Grip Dips: These are another variation of the dips that you can do with the bar in the same position. Instead of grabbing the rounded bars, this time you will grab the ends of the straight bar and lower yourself down and back up. This is a more difficult variation and focuses less on your arms and lats and more on your scapular rotators and depressors. Your feet can again be either straight or bent depending on your difficulty level.

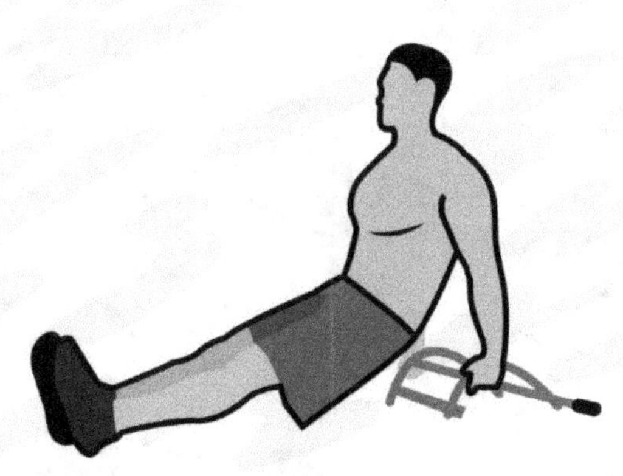

Incline Hammer Push-ups: Place the bar face down with the rounded parts up and hold on to the rounded bars. Place your feet together on the floor behind you and do a slow and controlled push-up. This is a great variation to your average push up because it puts your body on a slight incline which engages the lower pectorals more than a standard push-up. It also changes the orientation of your hands into a more supinated position which changes the recruitment of the triceps and elbow extensor muscles.

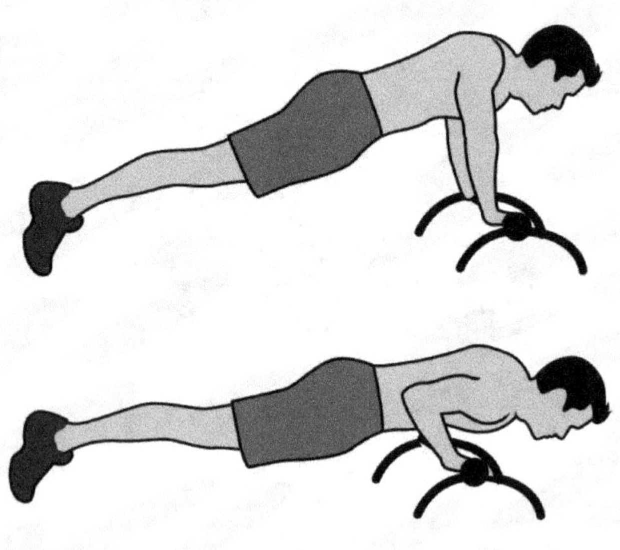

Wide Grip/Close Grip Incline Push-Ups: With the bar placed on the ground face down, you can also perform push-ups using the straight part of the bar. You can either hold the straight bar on the outer edge of the handles for wide grip or in between the rounded bars with your hands touching together for the close grip push-ups. Narrow grip push-ups are better for working your triceps as well as the inner part of your chest muscles. The wider grip push-ups are better for working the outer chest muscles and shoulder stabilizers.

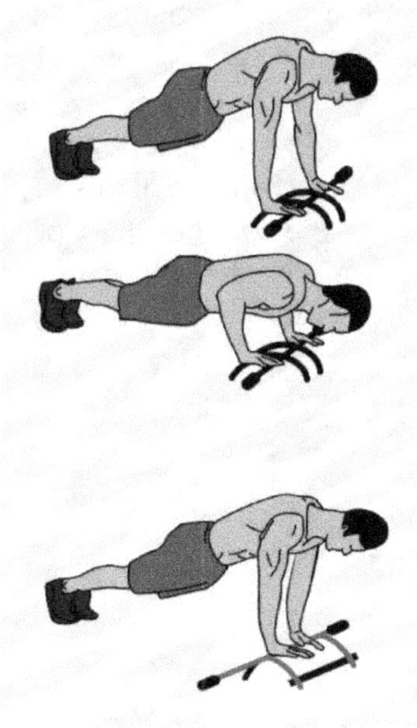

Incline/Decline Planks: Planks are another great way to work most of the muscles in your body. They work your muscles isometrically which is a great way to increase core stability. There are two different ways you can use your pull-up bar to do a plank. First place the bar on the ground face down. Then, you can start by placing your feet on the bar and your arms or elbows on the ground while you bring your body straight into the plank position and attempt to hold for 30-60 seconds. Make sure the bar is placed up against a wall, so it doesn't slide out from you during the exercise. These are called decline planks and will place a slightly greater emphasis on your back stabilizers and posterior shoulder muscles. With your elbow bent, your plank will be a much easier than with your arms straight. When your arms are straight, the plank will work not only your abdominals and back muscles, but your shoulder stabilizers and rotator cuff will be more engaged as well. You can also do the planks with your arms straight while grabbing the rounded part of the bar while your feet are on the ground. This variation is an incline plank and will place more emphasis your pectorals and anterior shoulder muscles.

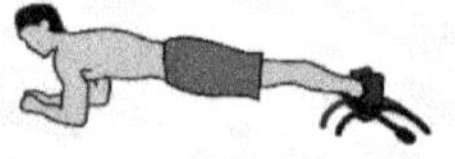 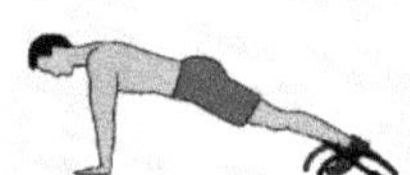 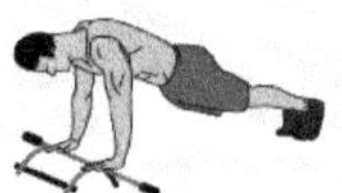

Mountain Climbs: Another exercise that you can perform with the bar on the ground is mountain climbs. They are not only an amazing exercise for your abdominals, but they are a great way to add some more cardio to your exercise routine. Just grab the top of the bar with your arms straight, then keep your body straight and core tight while you alternately bring your knees up towards your arms at as fast a pace as you can tolerate. The faster you go, the more cardiovascular exercise you will get out of it.

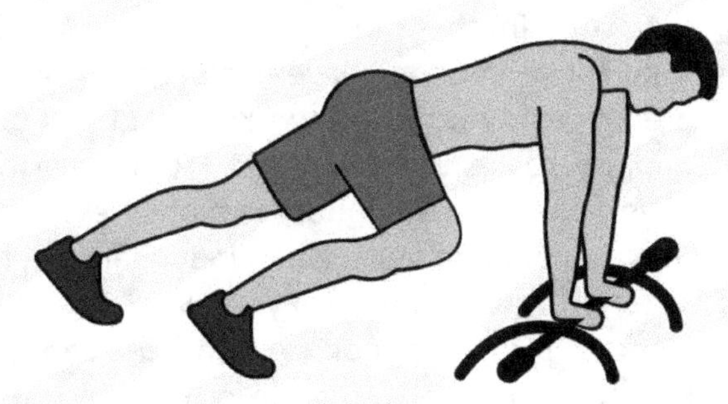

Overview of Workout Routines

Now that you have completed your first pull-up and have a good understanding of the other exercises listed, it is time to ramp things up and get the most out of your home pull-up bar. You are probably wondering how many sets and reps you should do once you get started. Don't worry, I will walk you through a basic workout routine and a then a more advanced routine that will be a little more difficult. The American Council on Exercise recommends performing 2-4 sets of 8-12 reps of pull-ups for optimal performance. This is a good baseline for starting a basic workout routine.

The following workout routines were developed by me from my experiences not only using doorway pull-up bars, but also from my work in the clinic as a physical therapist. I understand that these methods have not been formally tested, and that there are many different workout routines out there. These just happen to be the ones that I think are the most effective for everyone from beginners to higher level athletes. I have also found that depending on what your goals are, there are a couple of different ways to perform your workouts.

In general, if you are looking to build strength, then I recommend doing 4 sets of 7-10 reps before reaching your point of exhaustion. If you are looking to increase muscle growth, then I recommend performing 4-8 sets to muscle exhaustion with 1-2 minutes of rest between sets. Below I will break down a couple of workout routines that include a lot of the exercises we discussed along with how many sets and repetitions to perform. Remember that these can be modified depending on your level and whether your goals are strength or building muscle. The sets and repetitions are only an estimate to give you an idea of where to start. Also, if you find that you cannot do the full amount of sets or reps, then do what you can, and work your way up to the full routine.

My workout routines consist of 4 days with 4 different exercises each day, and 4 sets of each exercise, with a day of rest between each exercise day. I find that it is necessary to give your muscles a day to rest and rebuild before working them again. Sets should be performed in an alternating manner, so you do the first set of each exercise, then the second set, and repeat 4 times until you have done all the sets. You should also take 1-2 minutes of rest between sets. Feel free to mix and match other exercises into the routine if you prefer other exercise more than the ones I have listed. Also, you can increase or lower the number of sets or repetitions depending on your goals. Remember, these are guidelines and not routines you need to follow step by step, unless you want to.

Beginner Routine

Day 1:

- <u>Wide Grip Pull-ups with Legs Behind:</u>
  4 Sets to Exhaustion
- <u>Crunches:</u>
  4 Sets of 20 Reps
- <u>Dead Hangs:</u>
  4 Sets of 30-60 Seconds
- <u>Wide Grip Push-Ups:</u>
  4 Sets of 10 Reps

Day 2:

- <u>Close Grip Pull-ups with Legs in Front:</u>
  4 Sets to Exhaustion
- <u>Sit Ups:</u>
  4 Sets of 20 Reps
- <u>Chin Ups:</u>
  4 Sets of 10 Reps
- <u>Close Grip Push-ups:</u>
  4 Sets of 10 Reps

Day 3:

- <u>Negative Pull-ups:</u>
  4 Sets of 10 Reps
- <u>Incline Push-Ups:</u>
  4 Sets of 10 Reps
- <u>Neutral Grip Pull-ups:</u>
  4 Sets to Exhaustion
- <u>Planks with Elbows on Floor:</u>
  4 Sets of 30-60 Second Holds

Day 4:

- <u>Mixed Grip Pull-ups:</u>
  4 Sets to Exhaustion
- <u>Dips with Knees Bent:</u>

4 Sets of 10 Reps
- <u>Hanging Forearm Curls:</u>
4 Sets of 10 Reps
- <u>Knee Raises:</u>
4 Sets of 10 Reps

Advanced Routine

Day 1:

- <u>Pull-ups with Knees Up:</u>
  4 Sets to Exhaustion
- <u>Dips with Legs Straight:</u>
  4 Sets of 20 Reps
- <u>Hanging Shrugs:</u>
  4 Sets to Exhaustion
- <u>Planks with Arms Straight:</u>
  4 Sets of 1-2 Minute Holds

Day 2:

- <u>Weighted Pull-ups:</u>
  4 Sets to Exhaustion
- <u>Incline Planks with Arms Straight:</u>
  4 Sets of 1-2 Minute Holds
- <u>Hanging Leg Raises:</u>
  4 Sets of 20 Reps
- <u>Wide Grip Dips with Legs Bent:</u>
  4 Sets of 20 Reps

Day 3:

- <u>Towel Grip Pull-ups:</u>
  4 Sets to Exhaustion
- <u>Wide Grip Dips with Legs Straight:</u>
  4 Sets of 20 Reps
- <u>Knee Side Raises:</u>
  4 Sets of 20 Reps
- <u>L-Hangs with Rotations:</u>
  4 Sets of 20 reps

Day 4:

- <u>Single Arm Pull-ups:</u>
  4 Sets to Exhaustion
- <u>Toes to Bar:</u>
  4 Sets of 20 Reps
- <u>Mountain Climbs:</u>
  4 Sets to 100 Reps at a fast pace
- <u>Side to Sides:</u>
  4 Sets of 20 Reps

Summary

You should now have enough exercises to keep you busy for a while. If you can perform even half of these exercises, you are well on your way to having the body you want. Like I mentioned above, this can be the last piece of exercise equipment that you will ever need to purchase if you use it correctly. I hope that this guide has given you some new ideas to get the most out of it. If you are having trouble doing some of the exercises, don't be discouraged. Just go slow and stay within your means. Even performing just one pull-up is no small feat. So, take your time and work hard, and you will get to where you want to be before you know it. Enjoy!